Make Your Penis Bigger

Make Your Penis Bigger

A Guide to Penis Exercises
That Increase Size and Improve Erections

H.J. Maxwell

To order additional copies of this book, contact:
Xlibris Corporation
1-888-795-4274
www.Xlibris.com
Orders@Xlibris.com
26815

CONTENTS

Introduction 9

The Exercises 11

Nutrition 13

Exercise for the body 15

Exercise 1 17

Exercise 2 19

Exercise 3 21

Exercise 4 23

Exercise 5 25

Exercise 6 27

Exercise 7 29

Exercise 8 31

Exercise 9 33

Exercise 10 35

Exercise 11 37

Exercise 12 39

Exercise 13 41

Exercise 14 43

Exercise 15 45

Exercise 16 47

Exercise 17 49

Exercise 18 51

Dedication

This book is dedicated to my brother,
Bobby Mike Maxwell, 1954-2004.

Introduction

This book will show you how to exercise your penis similar to the way you can exercise any other part of your body. Improve your sex life and the way you feel about yourself as a man. Erections are improved as well. The results can be dramatic. Your progress will depend on your initial size, and the quality and consistency of your workouts.

The Exercises

We start with a series of stretching and toning exercises. Concentrate on contracting the area of the penis between your hands. In the beginning, when the muscles may be weak, the maximum contraction that can be achieved may not be great. This will improve with time. The exercises are most effective when the penis is flaccid, or not erect. The isometric warm up exercises will help you get a feel for how the dumbbell exercises should be done. The dumbbell or weight training exercises are where you can get some big increases in size, both length and thickness. They can also greatly improve erections.

I like to do two minutes of hand exercises followed by ten minutes of dumbbell work. Like other weight training, do these exercises every other day. The muscles will need time to rest and rebuild. I like to workout three days a week.

Nutrition

Proper nutrition is important in achieving and maintaining a healthy sex life. A well balanced diet of protein, carbohydrates, and fats forms the foundation. Maintain three to four servings a day of protein at all times. Cut back on carbohydrates and fats when you are trying to lose body fat. Supplements are good for added nutrition. The mineral zinc has been shown to increase the testosterone level. Drink plenty of water and try to get three to four servings of fruits and vegetables per day. Micro-nutrients from fruits and vegetables are now available in capsule form, Hold alcohol consumption down to a moderate level. Avoid nicotine for your own health and those around you.

Exercise for the body

Proper exercise of the body contributes to your physical, mental, and emotional well-being. Stretching, strength training, and aerobics are all important. I like to do a series of ten second stretches for versatility. With this method I am also able to get in a large variety of exercises in fifteen to twenty minutes. Strength training is a must for good health as we get older. The back must be kept strong and flexible in order to maintain vitality. The back supports the spine, which is an extension of the brain. I prefer dumbbells to start with because they are so versatile. Barbells and machines are a nice addition to your exercise program . Two to three minutes of stretching is a great way to relieve stress at the end of the day, and can add a great deal to your sex life.

Exercise 1

Hold the penis in both hands to isolate the middle area of the penis between the testicles and the tip .Grip the tip of the penis around the ridge firmly. Pull the penis with the hands and contract the area between the hands for ten to fifteen seconds if possible. Relax and repeat as desired.

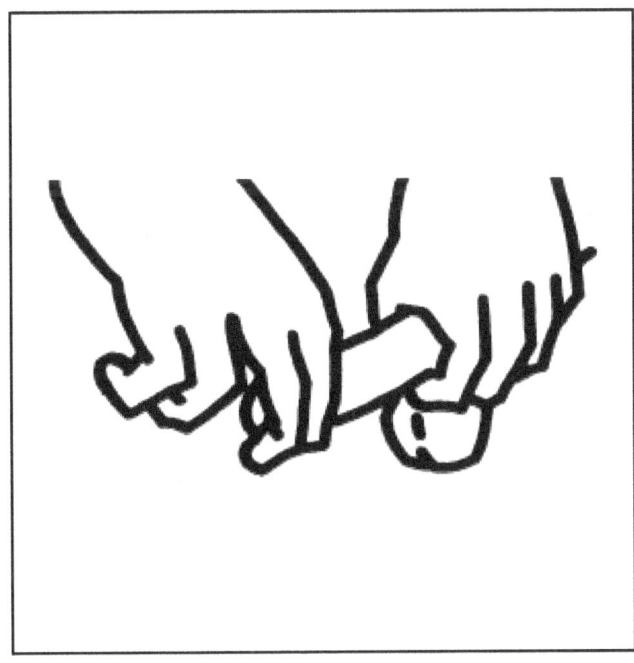

Exercise 2

Same procedure as exercise 1, however rotate the penis upside down.

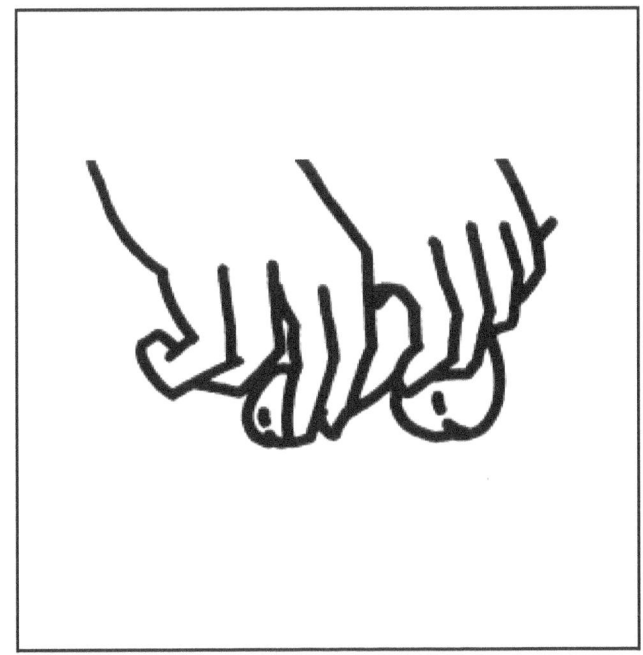

Exercise 3

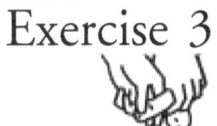

Same procedure as exercise 1, however rotate the penis to the side.

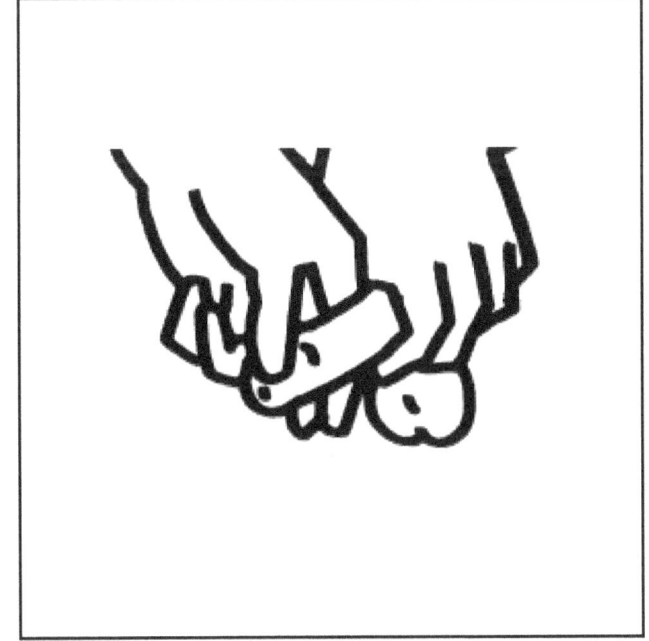

Exercise 4

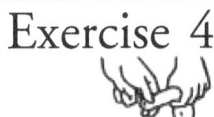

Same procedure as exercise 1, however rotate the penis to the other side.

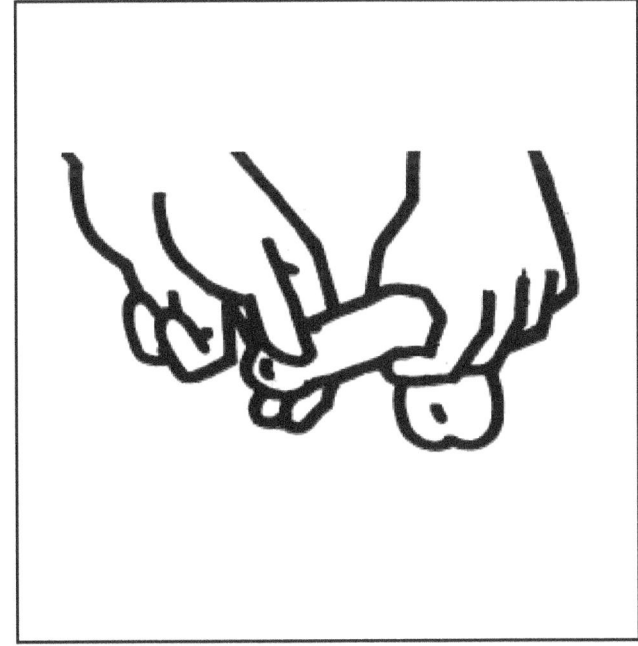

Exercise 5

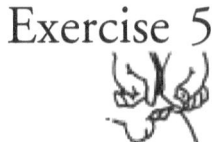

Hold the penis on the between the tip and middle of the penis. Contract the muscles in the area isolated by the fingers for ten to fifteen seconds if possible. Relax and repeat as desired.

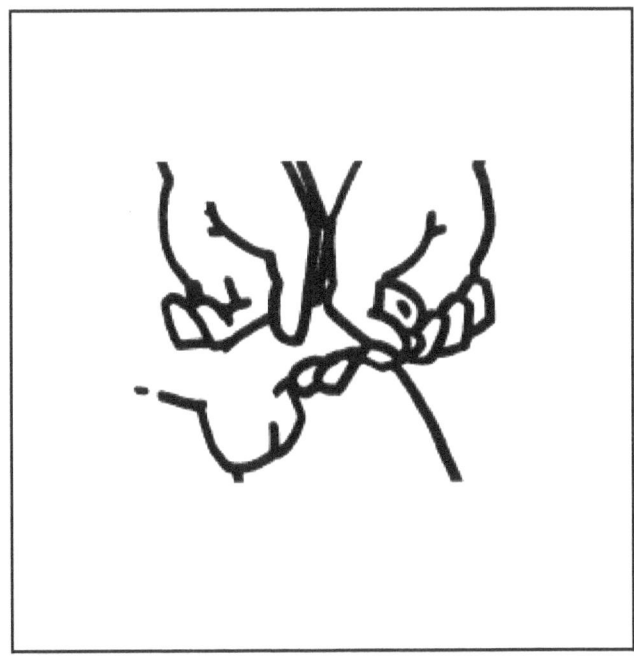

Exercise 6

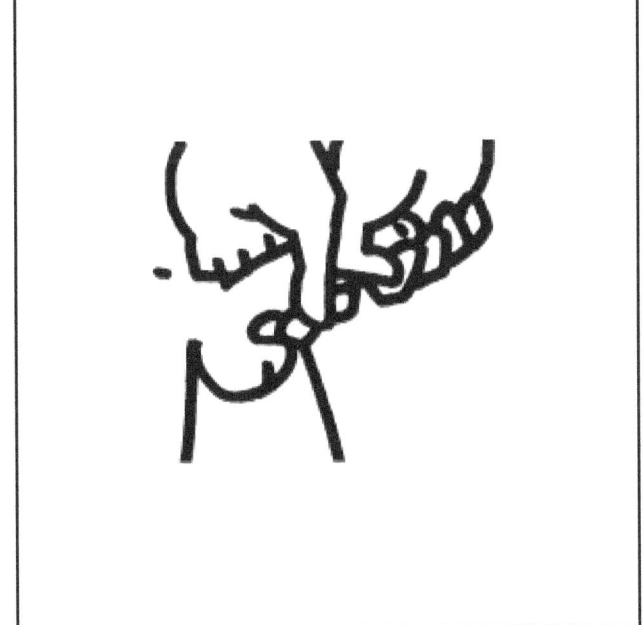

Same procedure as exercise 5, however rotate the penis upside down.

Exercise 7

Same procedure as exercise 5, however rotate the penis to the side.

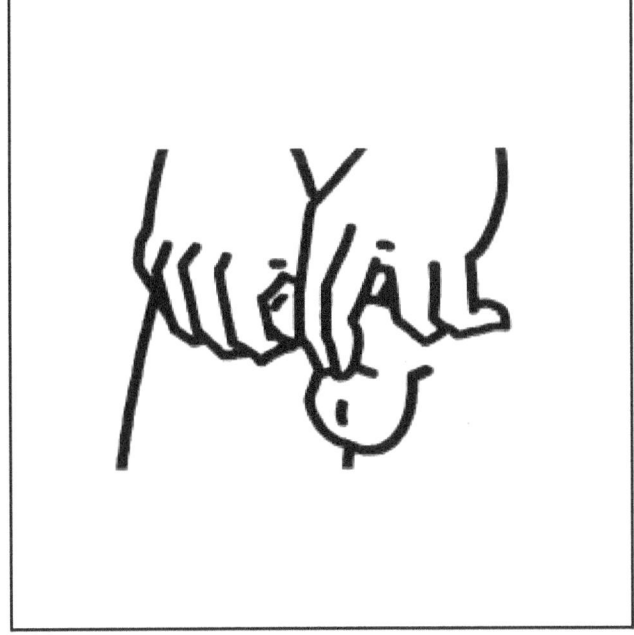

Exercise 8

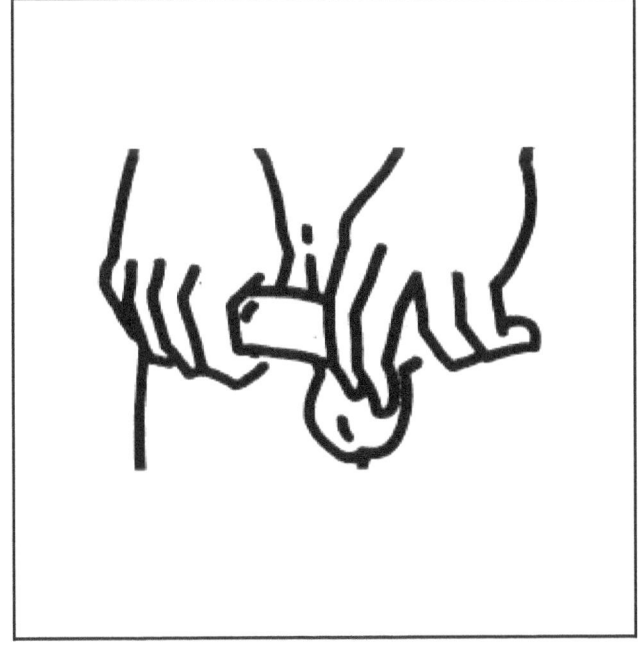

Same procedure as exercise 5, however rotate the penis to the other side.

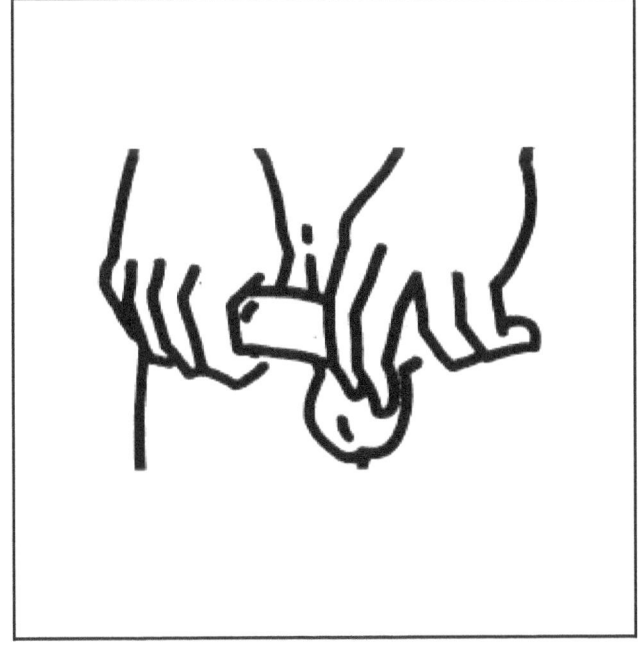

Exercise 9

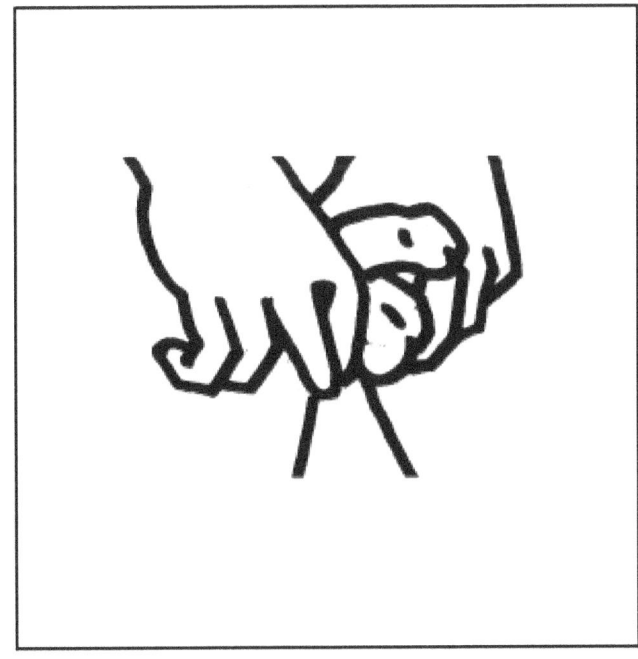

Hold the penis in both hands, just under and above the testicles. So as to isolate the part of the penis close to the body. Contract the muscles in this area for ten to fifteen seconds if possible. Relax and repeat as desired.

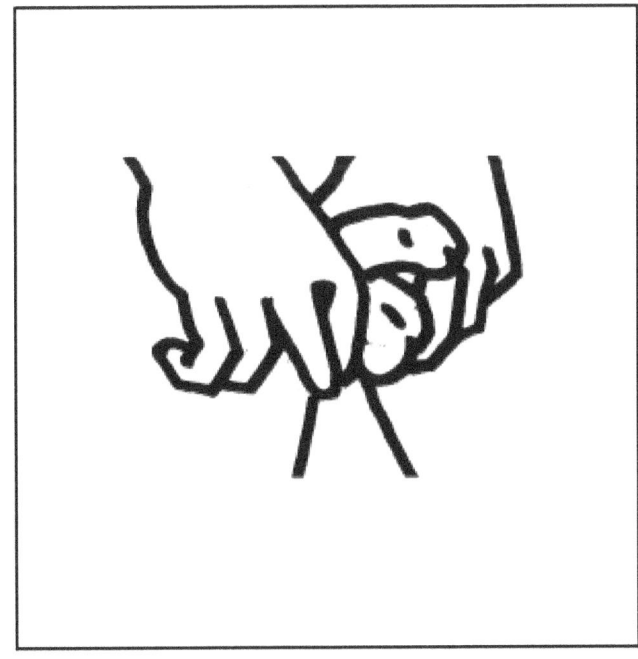

Exercise 10

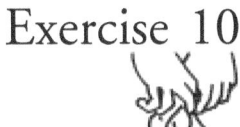

Same procedure as exercise 9, however rotate the penis upside down.

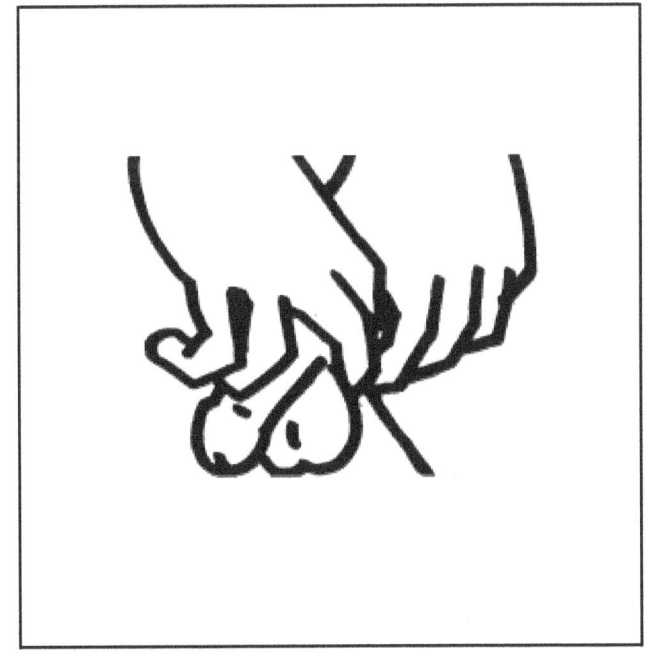

Exercise 11

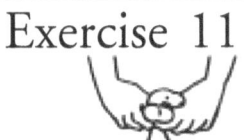

Same procedure as exercise 9, however rotate the penis to the side.

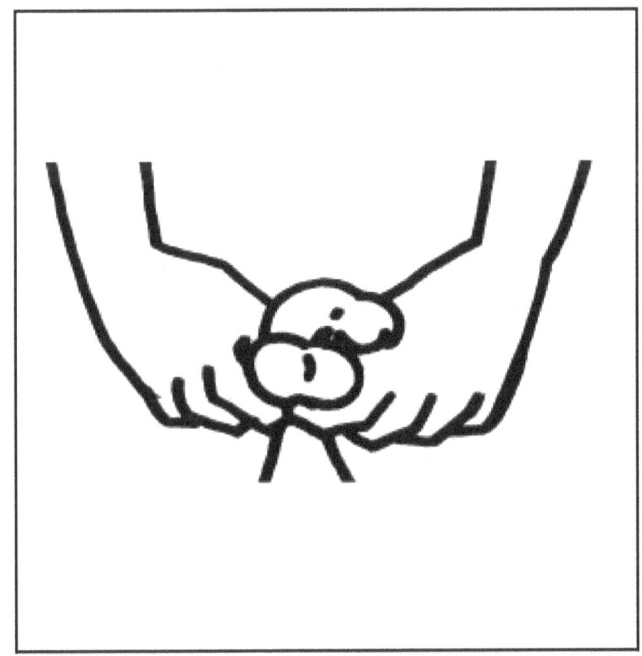

Exercise 12

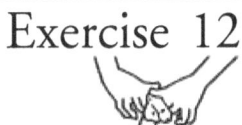

Same procedure as exercise 9, however rotate the penis to the other side.

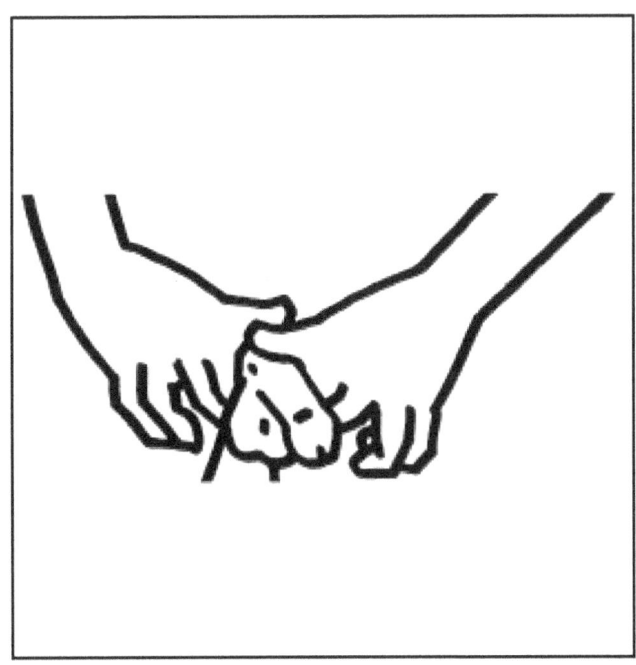

Exercise 13

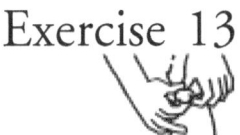

Hold the end of the penis with both hands using the fingertips. Contract the muscles in the head of the penis for ten to fifteen seconds if possible. Relax and repeat as desired.

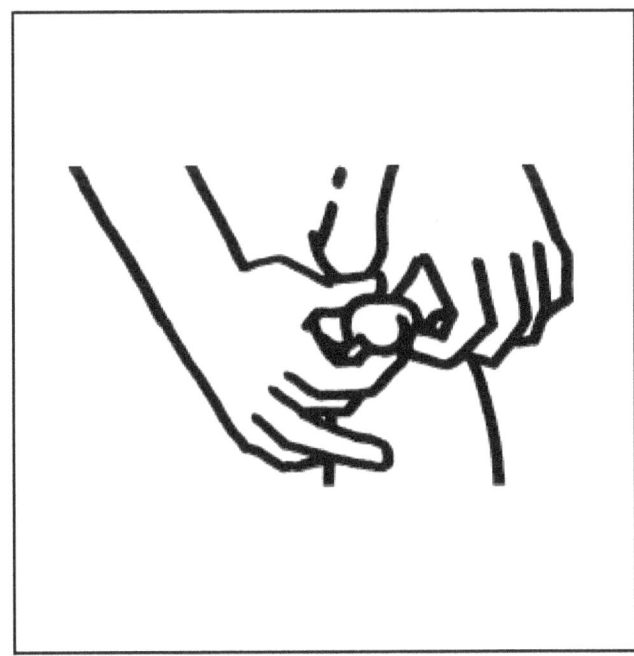

Exercise 14

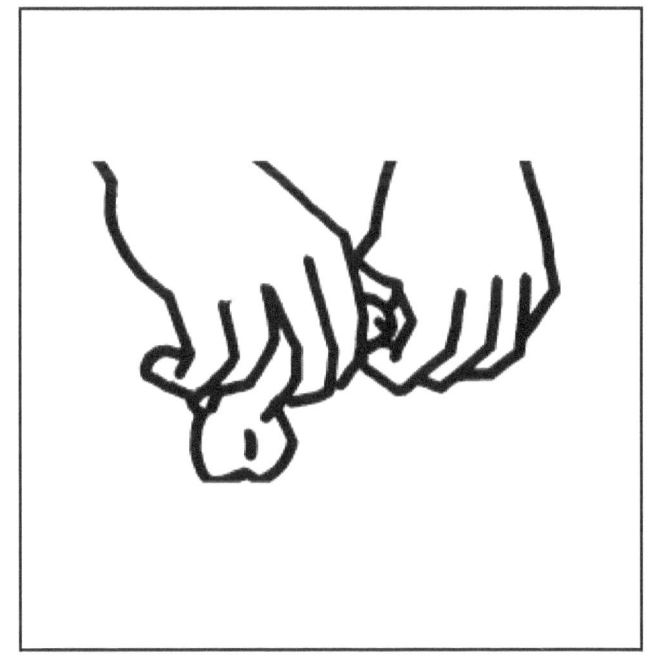

Same procedure as exercise 13, however hold the penis upside down.

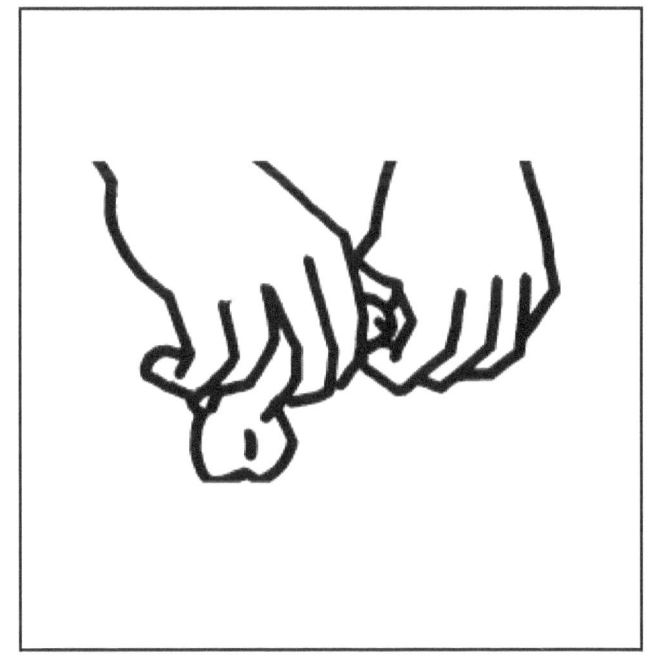

Exercise 15

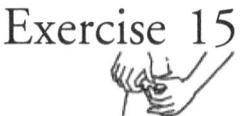

Same procedure as exercise 14, however rotate the penis to the side.

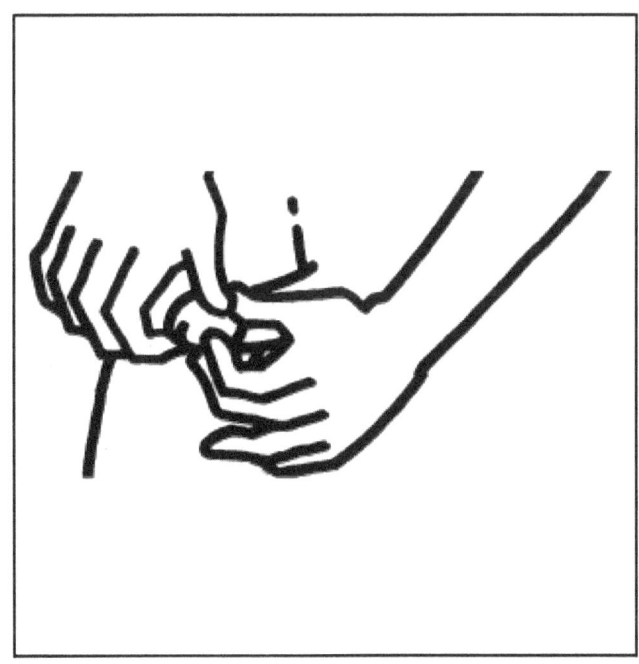

Exercise 16

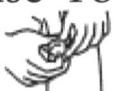

Same procedure as exercise 14, however rotate the penis to the other side.

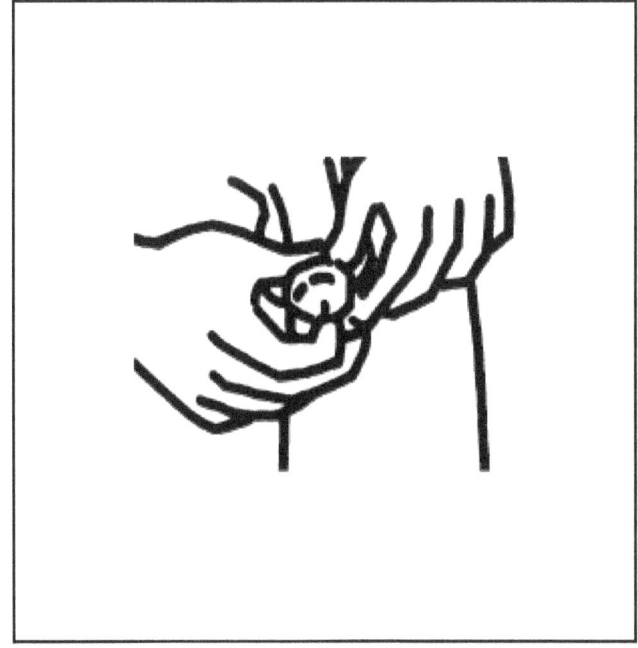

Exercise 17

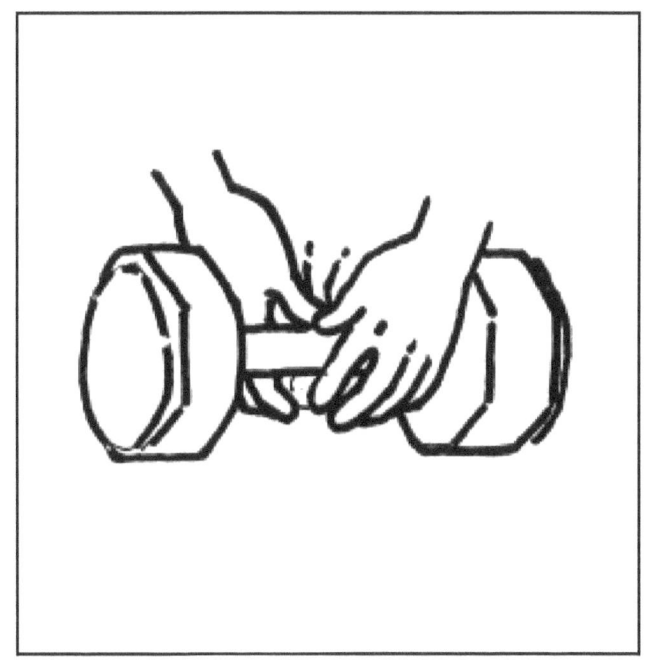

These exercises can be done with a stationary exercise bar or a dumbbell.

Exercise 18

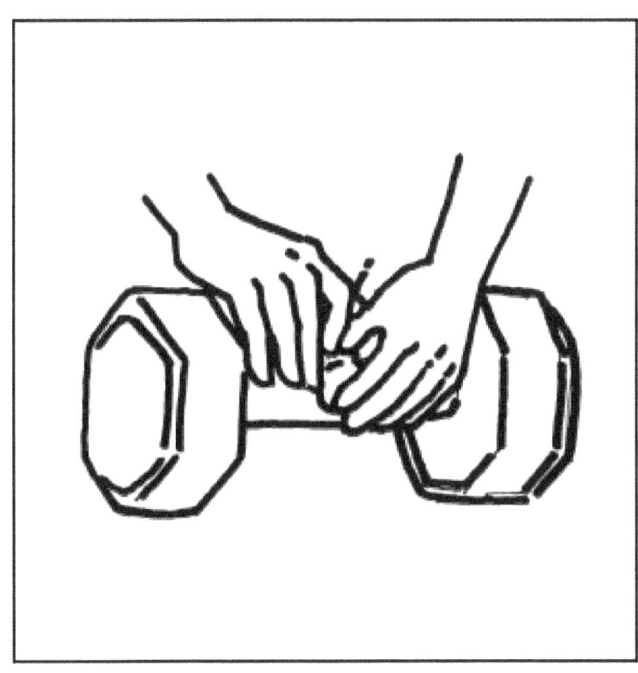

I prefer to place a dumbbell on a cabinet, bench or table about crotch high. I use a 35 pound hexagon weight. It is tall enough for me to reach under and remains completely stationary when doing the exercises. I place a bath cloth under the weight for stability. If the bar has a rough finish you will want to put a piece of tape on the bar for comfort. If you use a dumbbell be careful not to drop it. Hold the penis in different positions and contract the muscles as you press the penis against the bar. You can do this exercise holding the penis under the bar and/or over the bar. Work different areas of the penis from the tip of penis to the crotch. Rotate the penis clockwise and counter clockwise for variations. Typically, I will contract the muscles for 15 seconds. It will take 5 to 10 seconds to move to another position.

www.ingramcontent.com/pod-product-compliance
Lightning Source LLC
Chambersburg PA
CBHW061224280526
45784CB00006B/2616